A Guide to Assessing Your Newborn's Condition at Home

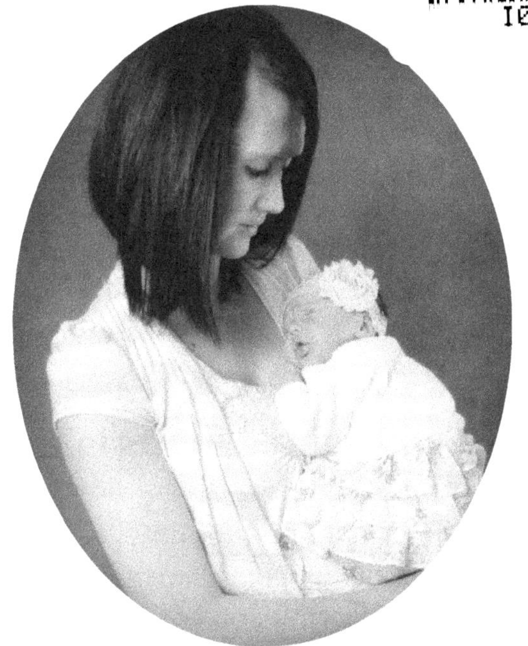

PHOTO BY LYNDSY

By Donna Young, ND
Traditional Midwife

Disclaimer

The information contained within this book is for educational purposes only. The information is not intended to replace available medical treatment nor is it intended to diagnose or treat disease. This information has not been approved by any entity, including the FDA.

Copyrighted material

The enclosed information is the intellectual property of the author. Do not copy any part of this book without the written permission of the author. No part of the material is to be copied or electronically saved.

Dedication

This book is dedicated to the wonderful ladies, and their husbands, who have gone the extra mile to insure the safety and well-being of their babies by faithfully putting forth the discipline of eating healthy, supplementing and exercising to get a more positive outcome in their pregnancies, births and babies.

A special thanks to Kaleb and Stephanie for encouraging this information be put in writing for every couple who may need it.

About the author

Donna Young is a Naturopathic trained traditional midwife with over 25 years of home birth experience, with an impressive success rate. Her line of expertise is female health, pregnancy and childbirth.

Donna is also the author of POWERFULLY PREGNANT, a system of prenatal care that allows women to be informed, healthy and in control of their own pregnancy while having a more positive outcome. Her ladies rave about their health and beauty during pregnancy as well as their shorter than average births and fewer complications. The health of mother and child are Donna's top priorities.

Table of Contents

Forward

Most new parents find themselves in a position where they are not sure what is 'normal' and what is not. Once baby is born, the parents are left with no real understanding what is within the ranges of normality. They may ask family members, friends, neighbors etc. and everyone has an opinion but they will inevitably conflict with each other and the most outspoken will generally be given credence whether their opinion is right or not. Most do not have a family member who has firsthand pediatric or newborn training so they go by what seems right to them, which may or may not be accurate. Other things might be over-looked or considered to be a family trait which really should be looked into more closely. This book will, hopefully, provide some direction.

There is a unique group of people who are choosing to do unassisted childbirth, this book is to give guidance to help them understand how to evaluate their own child and have a reference to help make decisions that are right for them and their child.

This book is intended to shed some light onto what a parent can look for in a newborn to have a more accurate analysis of how their baby is doing. It is for both pace of mind as well as some known indicators for needing additional help.

If there is any doubt as to how baby is doing then it is always best to err on the side of caution and have baby looked at by a care provider if possible.

Suggested things to have on hand

Cloth measuring tape

Stethoscope

Thermometer

Oximeter for infants

Bulb Syringe (3 ounce)

DeLee Suction Trap

Scales to weigh baby (digital bathroom scales work fine)

APGAR

APGAR is a method of scoring the condition of a newborn with a quick summary of a baby's signs at 1 minute, 5 minutes and sometimes 10 minutes after birth. The 10 minute check is done always if the 5 minute score is under "7".   However, this same guideline can be used to determine the wellbeing of a baby at any point because if they fall beneath the levels of normality then they need to be seen by a care provider directly.

APGAR stands for Activity, Pulse, Grimace, Appearance, and Respiration. Each category is given a rating of 0, 1 or 2 depending on the condition. A baby with an APGAR of 0 is non-responsive or "floppy". A perfectly healthy and strong baby in prime condition has an APGAR of 10. We would consider a baby with an APGAR score of "7" to be 70% of healthy, with 30% needed to be improved. All babies should have an APGAR of 10 within 10 minutes after their birth however an APGAR of 8 is acceptable as long as baby is making steady improvement.

The APGAR system is the fastest way to determine the over-all well-being of a newborn.

Here is how the point system for APGAR works.

Activity (Muscle tone)
Active, spontaneous movement with good muscle tone = **2 pts**.
Arms and legs flexed with little movement = **1 pt**.
No movement. "Floppy" tone = **0 pts**.

Pulse (Heart rate)
Normal (Heartbeat is over 100 beats per minute = **2 pts**
Heartbeat below 100 beats per minute = **1 pt**
Absent = **0 pts**.

Grimace (Facial reflexes)
Cough, sneeze = **2 pts**.
Facial grimace = **1 pt**.
No response = **0 pts**.

Appearance (skin color)
Pink or normal coloring all over body = **2 pts**.
Pink body with blue extremities = **1 pt**.
Blue, blue-gray, pale = **0 pts**.

Respiratory (breathing)
Good sustained cry, regular breathing = **2 pts**.
Slow, irregular, shallow breaths – **1 pt**.
Absent = **0 pts**.

If baby has a low APGAR of under 7, especially if the heart or lungs are involved, then baby needs to be seen by a professional immediately. Oxygen is generally given to assist with baby having support until the lungs and heart can function on their own.

At home births, generally baby is checked by APGAR first and then if baby is showing well (and there are no complications with mother or child) then they are given an opportunity to bond for a few minutes prior to having the rest of the newborn check done. In hospital births the baby is usually taken immediately by the nurses to do a check on baby while the doctor finishes delivering the placenta and cleaning mom up and then the family is allowed to bond afterward.

Babies can be born with a good APGAR and then have trouble holding their pink color or have trouble crying or the heart becomes irregular, even hours or days later. If any of these things happen then baby will need immediate attention. This is a reason for transport.

Cord

The umbilical cord is a network of vessels that contain one large vein, two smaller arteries, a very tiny vessel called a urachus and Wharton's jelly all bound together with a coating of an outer lining called Amniotic Epithelium. The umbilical cord takes nutrition and oxygen from the mother to the baby as well as taking the waste products from baby to the mother's kidneys.

The system is fairly simple. There are three vessels going through the umbilical cord. The vein is taking nutrition from the mother, through the placenta, to baby. The arteries take the waste products from the baby, back to the placenta, then to mother's kidneys and out of her body. The Wharton's Jelly is a gelatin type substance that holds the three vessels together to form a stronger cord instead of leaving them fragile, independent vessels.   The entire cord is usually about as thick as an average sized woman's little finger. Some are larger and some a little smaller. They vary in length from 7 inches to about 25 inches with the average being around 20-21 inches.

Usually a baby born with a 2 vessel cord (aka Single Artery Cord) is fine. However, a two vessel cord shows there is potential for baby to have either a kidney issue or a heart issue. Extra attention needs to be given to make sure baby does not have either of these problems. (For more information read the 'Kidney' and 'Heart' sections. When in doubt, talk to your care provider. If baby's APGAR is good then it should not be an emergency.

If a cord does not have Wharton's Jelly then one can see the open vessels independently without them being bound together as a cord and the vessels are left alone and weakened.

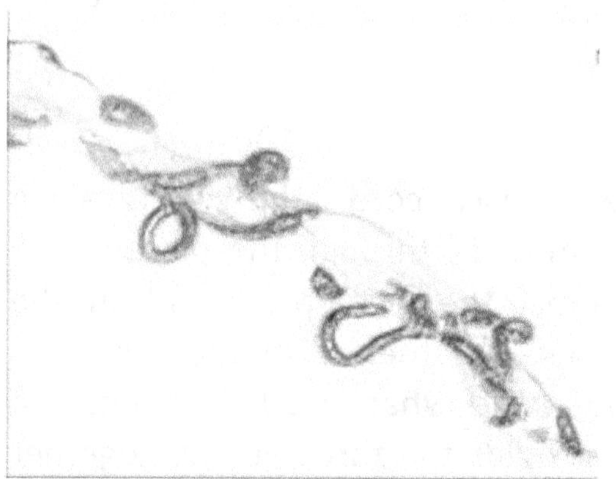

A lack of Wharton's Jelly can also lead to what is called a velamentous cord insertion. This is where the exposed vessels are attached to the placenta at a more surfaced level and does not have the support of the wharton's jelly to give the cord strength. Both of these conditions make the cord very weak which can lead to a lack of nutrition or waste removal during pregnancy or a hemorrhage or loss of life at the birth.

A lack of Wharton's Jelly says mother did not get enough nutritional support during pregnancy and the cord needs to be handled very gently to avoid having any of the vessels break while the cord is still attached to baby or mother. The breaking of a vessel, if the cord still has circulation, could cause a hemorrhage with either mother or child. In the event of an assisted birth then the attendant would know how to handle it. If this is an unassisted birth, then extra caution must be used to not pull on the cord and placenta should be allowed to deliver spontaneously after the cord is cut to secure baby.

Cry

Baby's cry should be strong, without fluid, grunts or chirps, with a clear air exchange. Most babies cry for several minutes after they are born and this is normal. Some babies will cry for less than 30 seconds and then lay and look around at their new surroundings, which is also OK as long as their color is good and their eyes are alert. These babies will generally have reasonably high APGARs.

The purpose of a cry is for baby to increase oxygen into their system to help adjust their lungs and heart to their new environment. Often a baby will have blue hands or feet and then cry until the extremities get ample circulation and turn pink then they stop crying on their own. If a one hushes a baby and tries to comfort it by stopping the crying, it interferes with this natural process. Babies should be allowed to cry for several minutes, a few times per day, to allow for the strengthening of the heart and lungs to keep baby healthy. A baby's cry is not out of emotion. Baby is not 'sad' or 'hurt' or 'afraid', directly after birth, but instead baby is acclimating to the new surroundings. This does not mean that a baby should never be comforted, but rather given them a few minutes to build their oxygen supply before soothing them, if they are not in a hurt or dangerous situation.

If fluid can be heard in the throat when baby cries, the care provider will usually use a bulb syringe or DeLee to clear the throat. The fluid generally comes from swallowing amniotic fluid during the birth and is cleared out in just a few minutes. This is usually done while baby is laying on it's side so gravity pulls the fluid to the bottom and allows for oxygen passage on the top. Once the fluid is gone then all is well and usually the issue is over with. If it needs to be done several times then it is not a problem as long as there is no blood or any other contributing factors such as fever or illness which warrant baby being seen by a professional.

When a baby has a weak cry then it is reason for concern. They can be preterm, with lungs or heart not fully developed. All babies should have a strong cry and should cry several times per day. If one has a 'really good baby' that 'never' cries then one may want to check the heart and lungs and check baby's oxygen level with an infant oximeter (such as an owlet or one from the local pharmacy). Other signs can be seen in the 'heart' and 'lung' sections. If things do not change shortly then baby should be seen by a care provider to make sure there is not a bigger problem.

If baby cries often and seems inconsolable but color is good then it is probably not life threatening but something is making baby uncomfortable such as pain in some area of the body, baby is not getting enough to eat, but once the problem is located then the crying should stop. As babies get older then they will pick up different cries such as hurt cry, angry cry, sick cry etc and the parents will learn to tell them apart.

There is also a system called the Dunstan Baby Language that could be looked into for the days and months following the birth. Very insightful regarding the way babies communicate.

Determining gestational age

When baby is in the womb, baby is covered with a soft white / cream colored waxy substance called vernix. Vernix is a protective coating to keep the skin from drying during exposure to the amniotic fluid. When a baby is born early term, there will be a substantial amount of vernix on baby. It will cover the entire body, head, legs, back stomach etc. and it is quite thick but wipes off easily with a cloth or paper towel.

When baby is near term, the vernix is all gone except under the arms, behind the knees and ears, and anyplace where the skin has folds.

When a baby is post term, then the vernix is completely gone and the skin is dry and can be cracked. Usually a little olive oil rubbed into the skin helps moisten the skin but it tells a person that baby was born after their actual due date.

The skin on an early-term baby will be thin and almost transparent. A baby born at or near due date will have a more red tint to the color with the skin looking thicker. The post term baby will be born with skin that is pink but it will be more cracked. The farther past the due date a baby is, the more cracked and dry the skin is.

With their posture, a baby born early-term will generally carry their legs and arms out straight because they have not been bound into a confined space like a full term or post term baby has been. A baby born at or near their due date will have a slight bend to their legs and a post term baby will have the knees tucked up and bent outwards and the arms will be bent. This happens when baby is out of room and has adapted to the more confined space in utero.

LEGS NEAR TERM   LEGS POST TERM

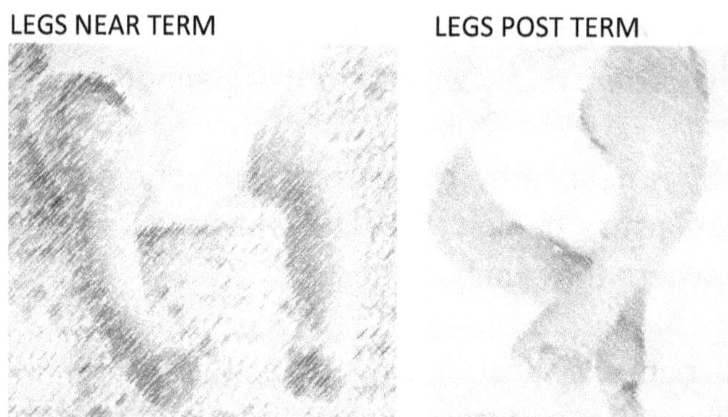

The fingernails on a baby that is post term will generally be longer than those of a near or early-term baby.
A preterm and early-term baby will have fewer creases on their hands and feet than one that is more

developed. Those will generally fill in with a little time.

Weight

Babies are weighed shortly after birth. The average weight of a full term newborn is about 7.5 lbs. Some are a little bigger and some are a little smaller, however, any weight between 5lbs and 10 lbs is considered normal.

Having baby scales is great but if those are not available then baby can be weighed on digital bathroom scales by having someone stand on the scales (on a hard floor like tile or linoleum—not on carpet) with a small blanket or towel in hand and get that weight. Then have that same person hold naked baby, in the towel or blanket and re-weigh. The difference between the two weights should be the size of the baby. This can be done with regular bathroom scales but it is not as accurate as the digital scales.

If mom was exposed to toxins, such as air pollution, then baby can weigh less. Other contributing factors can include poor diet, genetics and baby being preterm or early-term. If baby weighs less than 5lbs it is considered LBW (Low Birth Weight) then baby needs to be watched closely, usually under the supervision of a professional. (This can be done with regular bathroom scales, but digital are more accurate).

Underweight babies are prone to have some problems that are less common in babies that have more size.   One problem they are prone to is under developed lungs. If the lungs are not fully developed they will have a difficult time crying and they may have a chirp or grunt when they try to cry. If this happens then baby needs to be transported immediately.

Another problem that smaller babies are prone to is difficulty latching on and nursing. Their mouths are a little smaller and it may be difficult to get a good latch. The muscles in their jaws are also weaker so they tire easily when nursing. If this is a problem then bottle feeding (with either mother's milk or formula) might be a solution however, they need regular feedings and it is important that nutrition starts shortly after birth and the weight needs to be watched that baby is not losing weight. Yes, it is normal for a baby to lose a few ounces during the first couple days prior to the mother's milk coming in but that needs to be minimized.

If babies are born in the 6lb to 8lb range then they are prone to have developed organs and able to latch on. Some need a little encouragement but they are usually capable of doing it.

Over weight babies have to work harder to be born. They are more prone to shoulder dystocia (baby's chest/shoulders are too wide for mom's pelvis so the get hung up during delivery) and it generally takes more effort from mom to pass baby through the birth canal.   Once they are born, they are prone to have low blood sugar and need to be watched closely that they actually eat and not fall asleep while trying to nurse. But they are tired after the birth and sleep a lot and need to be encouraged to eat, especially if it was a longer birth

All babies should be re-weighed a couple times a week to insure baby is still gaining and a chart kept for the parent's own records.

When babies are born at 7.5 lbs or lighter, the skin can be loose and appear to be wrinkled. As baby gains weight then the skin and muscle will fill in and a visual of baby's skin and muscle will show baby is either gaining or losing weight. Given a little time the legs should start looking thicker and develop little rolls. See growth charts (pages 21-22) for the normal ranges one would expect to see in baby development.

If baby is dehydrated the fontanel (baby's soft spot) can be sunken in and the skin will become dry and there will be less urine output and thicker stools. There can be other signs baby is losing weight and needs to be watched closely. Vomiting, sweating, diarrhea, will all cause dehydration and little ones dehydrate quickly so it is important that they be watched closely and if there is any signs of weakness or lethargy then they need to be seen by a care provider directly, where they would usually be given electrolytes.

Length

Baby is measured from the top of the head to the flat of the heel when leg is gently stretched out. The average length of a baby is 18-22 inches. If a baby is longer than 22 inches, it is usually either from genetics or from being post term. Check the other signs of baby being an older gestational age before chalking it up to genetics.

If baby is shorter than 18 inches, then baby can be either early or have genetics on one side of the family that account for the length. Something that can cause a shorter length is a possible failure to thrive situation where, for whatever reason, baby did not get enough nutrition and if that is the case then it is important that baby be watched closely. If baby is early then not only will it be shorter but it will also be accompanied by a lighter birth weight.

Over the next few weeks, baby will put on more length as well as weight. Keeping a record of baby's growth can tell how they are progressing and is always nice to include in their chart or their baby book. Keeping record of this may also be needed in the future for their doctor or the State, if needed, as well as a keepsake. Records are always a good thing. Growth charts assist in tracking weight.

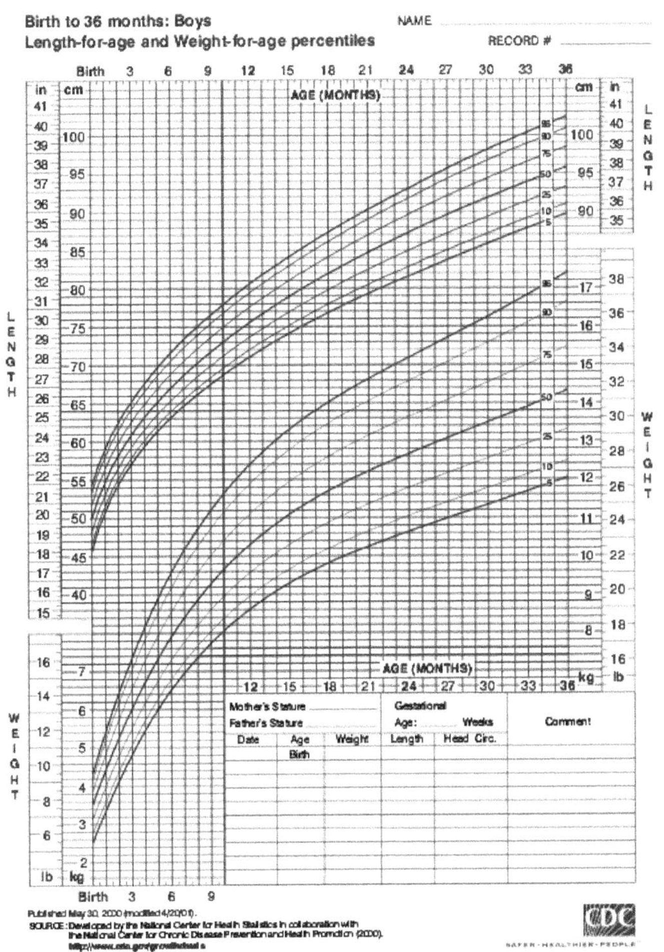

Birth to 36 months: Boys
Length-for-age and Weight-for-age percentiles
NAME
RECORD #
Birth 3 6 9 12 15 18 21 24 27 30 33 36
AGE (MONTHS)
in cm
41
40 100
39
38 95
37
36 90
35
34 85
33
32 80
31
30 75
29
28 70
27
26 65
25
24 60
23
22 55
21
20 50
19
18 45
17
16 40
15
LENGTH
cm in
100 40
39
38
95 37
36
90 35
LENGTH
95
90
75
50
25
10
5
38
17
36
16
34
15
32
14
30
13
28
12
26
WEIGHT
95
90
75
50
25
10
5
16
7
14
6
12
5
10
4
8
3
6
2
lb kg
WEIGHT
AGE (MONTHS)
12 15 18 21 24 27 30 33 36 kg lb
11 24
10 22
9 20
8 18
16
Mother's Stature
Father's Stature
Gestational
Age: Weeks
Comment
Date   Age   Weight   Length   Head Circ.
Birth
Birth 3 6 9
Published May 30, 2000 (modified 4/20/01).
SOURCE: Developed by the National Center for Health Statistics in collaboration with
the National Center for Chronic Disease Prevention and Health Promotion (2000).
http://www.cdc.gov/growthcharts
CDC
SAFER · HEALTHIER · PEOPLE

CDC GIRLS GROWTH CHART

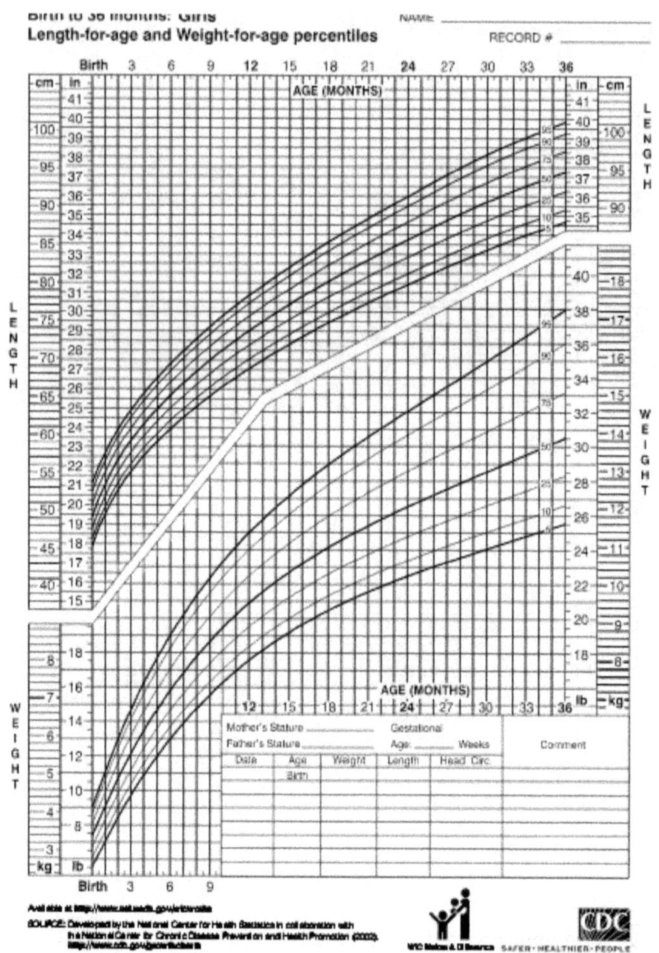

Head Circumference

The next measurement is the size of the head. With a cloth measuring tape, gently measure around the full part of baby's head. This measurement is done above the eyebrow and above the ears.

On a baby that is early, this measurement could be about 12 inches. Near term or term babies (6-7.5 lbs.) will generally have a 13-14 inch head. Post term or bigger babies may have a 15 inch head. Diet can also play a role in the size of the head.

Baby's head will be more round if baby spent a small amount of time in the birth canal or was delivered by c-section. While babies who had a long push time, may have a pointed or misshaped head or have a fluid swelling on the head at the pressure point which usually subsides in a few days or weeks. If there is any bruising or discoloration then baby needs to be seen by a care provider.

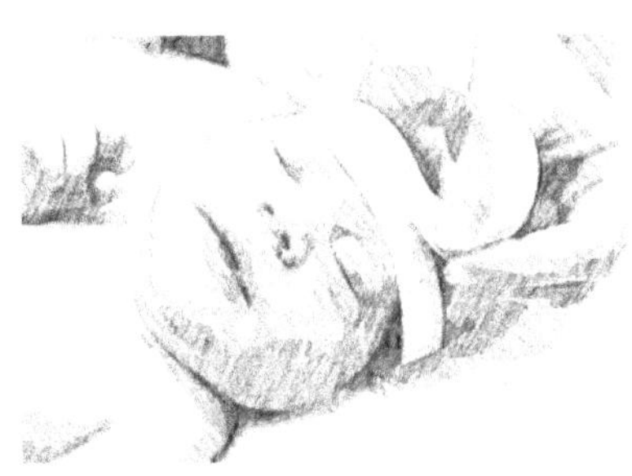

Fontanels

The fontanels are the soft spots on baby's head. When baby was developing, the skull was formed in flexible plates that slide together to allow baby to pass down through the birth canal with less stress on mother or child. Another purpose for this is to allow room in the skull for the brain to grow and develop without restriction. They will gradually fill in with bone over the coming months, the back one in 2-3 months and the top one in about 18 months.

The anterior fontanel is on top of baby's head and is diamond shaped with the points going front to back, to connect with the posterior fontanel, and cross-way running down to each temple. A pulse can been seen or felt in the top one if gently touched. The fontanel is supposed to be pretty close to even with the top of the skull. If it is sunken, it can show dehydration, so make sure baby is getting enough to drink. If it is bulging and raised up then it generally shows there is pressure inside the skull. This can happen when baby cries but if it also stays that way when baby is calm then baby should been seen by a professional to determine if there is an underlying problem such as a virus, or excess fluid on the brain.

The posterior fontanel is triangular shaped and is smaller than the top one and is found on the back of the head. This one is far more subtle, and not as notable as the top one.

Eyes

The eyes should be alert, focused and able to follow something when it moves. A baby should have near sighted vision capabilities at birth. They see from the moment they are born but sometimes need to have them cleaned off with a clean towel or cloth and they look around the room at different objects and people. The first time baby gets the opportunity to look at the mother, they will gaze into the mother's eyes. When baby hears another familiar voice then they will often turn to put a face with the voice. A newborn's eyes are very sensitive to bright light, so dimming the light or casting a shadow over baby's eyes help baby to focus better.

The eyes should be even. They should be at the same level, shaped the same and placed similar to one or both of the parents. When the eyes move, they should move smoothly without jerks and they should be able to focus on who is holding them. The eyes should not be crossed, but point in the same direction when they are looking at anything. If there is a problem that does not improve over the next few weeks then they will probably need to be seen by an eye doctor.

The eyes should not have goo or discharge in them and the lids should not be red or inflamed. There should not be any kind of infection. If there is any kind of discharge then they can be wiped with a clean, warm, damp cloth. If it seems there is infection then baby will need to be seen by a care provider sooner than later. It is not a matter of run to the ER but more watch closely and if you are not getting ahead of it then get hold of someone who can keep it from worsening. Never let infections worsen before getting help.

Newborn babies do not, generally, have tears until they are older. There are no tears to help wash out infections and there are no tears with crying. Usually babies develop tears between 2 weeks and two months after birth.

Bulging eyes can show pressure on the brain or a possible thyroid issue and warrant baby being seen by a professional, especially if the bulging is accompanied with pain (excess crying), bruising or lethargy.

Ears

The ears should be fully developed and placed at a level where the top of the ear is above the corner of the eye. If baby has down syndrome, the top of the ear will set below the corner of the eye. If baby does have down syndrome then there will be other signs as well such as fewer lines in the palms of the hands and feet, smaller hands, and a flattened facial profile including the cheek bones and nose.

If part of the outside of the ear is missing then it is called Anotia and if the entire external part of the ear is missing then it is called Microtia. These would be obvious at the birth and baby should be seen by a care provider within the next few days if possible.

The State would like all babies to have a hearing test to exclude the possibility of deafness. Some parents feel they do not want to have the testing done, for a variety of reasons from religious to financial. So with those parents, they check their own child with a couple of techniques. One is to watch to see if baby responds to the voice of someone talking to them or whistles or other tones. Secondly, generally, hearing babies will sleep through the light being turned on when they are sleeping, while non-hearing babies will wake immediately with the light being turned on. When in doubt, have them checked. This is not something that needs to be done immediately but should be done within the weeks after the birth.

Nose

Baby should be able to breathe through the nose without the assistance of mouth breathing. When baby is resting, the mouth should be closed and breathing just through the nose. During breastfeeding, baby should be able to nurse without have to take breaks away to catch breath.

By listening, one should be able to tell if there is fluid in the nasal passages. If there is then it can easily be cleaned out with a DeLee or bulb syringe.

If baby cannot breathe just through the nose then there are several things it can be. 1) The most common is amniotic fluid in the nose or mouth from being born. 2) If baby has a weak heart then they will breathe through the nose and mouth together, but this is usually accompanied with blueness of the hands, feet and around the mouth as well as having a weak cry or not cry much at all. (See more in the heart section.) 3) Very rarely it can be something is blocking the passages like a birth defect or a cyst etc.

If the parents have done what they can and baby is not breathing through the nose then the baby should be seen by a care provider.

Mouth

The mouth is looked at to make sure it is complete and without a harelip (aka a cleft lip). A harelip is a gap in the lip, up towards the nose. A clean or gloved pinkie is inserted into the mouth with the pad of the finger upward towards the roof of the mouth, at which time baby will generally begin to suck. This tells the strength of the suction and if baby has the strength to nurse and extract nutrition from the mother's breast. It also gives a chance to feel if there is a hole in the roof of the mouth. The hole would be called a cleft pallet, which is a birth defect that prevents baby from getting suction and being able to nurse. This warrants having baby seen within the first few hours after birth.

The next thing is to look and see if the mouth is shaped the same on both sides of the face. Does one side droop? Does one side not move when baby cries? This would show potential for a possible stroke and warrants medical attention.

When baby is relaxed, can baby breathe through the nose with the mouth closed completely? If not, then the gaping of the mouth is baby breathing through the mouth in order to get more oxygen than they are comfortable with the mouth closed. This can be because of a blockage in the nasal passage, which will show as baby making noise through the nose when they are breathing. If there is no nasal noise then it is more likely being caused by a weakening in baby's heart.

Skull

The skull should be uniformly shaped on all sides. There should not be malformations. The skull has two fontanels and suture lines that form the plates together. Immediately after birth the sutures generally overlap a little from the pressure of a vaginal birth but those should smooth out in the first hours after birth. On occasion there will be a little fluid spot between the skull and the skin, this is from the pressure of a vaginal birth and generally goes away in a few days. If it was a long or difficult birth then it could take up to a few weeks to go down. If the swelling seems in excess or if there is bruising associated with it then baby should be seen by a professional. If the bone itself is misshaped then baby should be seen by a care provider. This is especially true if the vision or eye movement is affected or baby is not able to nurse.

Heart

A stethoscope is used to check baby's heart. If one is not available, then one can gently put their ear to baby's back or chest to hear the heartbeat. The heart should be listened to for a full 60 seconds to get an understanding of what is happening.

A newborn baby's heart rate should be about 140 bpm (beats per minute). Rates that are anywhere between 100 to 160 bpm are considered normal. It can dip down to 90 when sleeping or up to 170 when under stimulation (crying). The resting rate would be about 35 beats in 15 seconds. If the heartbeat, stays outside of a normal range, then it warrants having baby seen by a care provider.

The rhythm of the heartbeat is as important as the number of beats per minute. You want to listen to the rhythm and make sure there is a regular rhythm without doubled or skipped beats. If there is an irregular heartbeat then baby should be seen by a care provider.

Other signs of a possible heart condition are blueness of the fingers, toes or around the mouth, shortness of breath or inability to cry, shortness of breath when laying on the stomach or left side and baby breathing through the nose and mouth together with mouth gaped open. For this reason, newborns should not be put down to sleep on their stomach, nor on the left side. And if baby is exhibiting 2 or more of the symptoms then one may want to have baby checked. If a baby has some blue or purple coloring, then usually it will clear up when baby cries. If baby has a strong cry then they oxygenate their own body and the color will lose the blue / purple tone.

Lungs

The lungs are listened to with either a stethoscope or an ear to the back. There is enough space taken out of the left lung to make room for the heart so the left lung is smaller. When listening to the lungs there should be a sound of clear air flow with each breath. There should be no crackling or wheezing. On each side we listen to the upper, middle and lower sections of the lung, where clear air exchange should be heard with each breath.

Sometimes when baby is born, they will swallow or inhale a little amniotic fluid which will end up in the throat and sometimes into the bronchial tubes (the tubes going from the nose and throat to the lungs). When this happens it is usually suctioned out with a bulb syringe from the throat, or a DeLee Suction Trap, which goes a little deeper. Baby can usually manage to keep the fluid out of the lungs by coughing and sneezing but occasionally it falls into the bronchials. If that happens then it will sound like crackling in the lung area when listened to. If there is crackling or wheezing that does not improve then baby should be seen as it can build into pneumonia. The concern is greater if there was meconium stain in the amniotic fluid at birth, due to potential for infection being greater.

Coughing and sneezing are normal for a newborn as this is their natural reflex to clear the sinuses and bronchials of any fluids acquired during birth. However, those fluids should be cleared out within the first couple of days after birth. If there are any fluids that cannot be cleared with a bulb syringe or DeLee, especially if the fluids are inhibiting breathing then baby should be seen by someone.

On occasion, a baby will have a movement while still in utero causing the amniotic fluid to be stained green. This warrants watching the baby closely for respiratory issues and may also cause baby to spit-up mucous in the first day or two after the birth as the body tries to get rid of it. This is normal but baby might need to be suctioned with a bulb syringe to assist in getting rid of the fluid. If there is fluid heard in the bronchials or lungs then baby needs to be seen by a care provider immediately to avoid having the fluid turn to pneumonia or infection. As long as it is not heard in the chest then it is fine to allow baby to clear it out naturally with the assistance of using a bulb syringe.

Rib cage

The rib cage, when measured at nipple level, should measure within ½ inch of the same size as the head circumference. If the chest is significantly smaller, then one wants to check for other signs of 'failure to thrive' of baby being malnourished and also check for signs of extra fluid on the head. If the chest is significantly larger, then one wants to check for other signs that may indicate a virus that may affect the forming of the head and brain, such as Zika. If there is more than an inch difference then baby may need to be seen by a professional.

The rib cage should not have any disfigurement. It should be uniform on both sides and it should allow room for the organs. Occasionally a baby is born with a 'sunken chest', which is where the sternum and rib cage are sunken in. As long as baby has a healthy cry then it should be fine because the lungs and heart have room to move and as the child matures then the protein consumption increases and the muscle should develop and pull the rib cage back into place. If the condition prevents baby from having a solid and healthy cry then it could imply that pressure may be being applied to the lungs and heart and baby may need to be seen by a professional.

Abdomen

When checking the abdomen, we first look at the naval, where the cord is inserted into the body, and by gently feeling around the outer side we look for any bulging that would suggest a herniation. If there is a hernia then baby will need to be seen by a professional at some point but most doctors will hold off until baby is 2-3 years old before doing surgery so it is not a rush.

The next thing we do is gently palpate (feel) across all areas of the abdomen for any kinds of lumps, swellings or painful areas within the abdominal cavity. If it is painful then baby will object to having it touched and may cry but not always. If any of these conditions happen then baby should be seen.

Intestinal sounds

While at the abdomen, put a stethoscope to the abdomen in all four sections and make sure you can hear gurgling. The gurgling says that baby's intestines are moving and baby is capable of having a bowel movement. If there is no gurgling and no bowel movements then baby will need to be seen by a care provider in the next day or two.

Hands

While looking at the hand we are not just counting fingers but also look at the color. There should be a healthy color all the way to the fingertips. If there is any blue or purple then it should go away when baby cries.

One wants to also notice the lines on baby's hands. Most babies have several lines and creases across the palms of the hands. If a child has Down's Syndrome then they will have a single line across the palm combined with a shorter and wider hand along with shorter fingers. This is not a reason to find outside help at this point.

Spine

Turning baby over onto it's side and looking at the back, we look for any bulging, bumps or any other irregularities in the spine. This is the time to observe for signs of spina bifida which is where the spinal cord shows on the outside of the body. This warrants baby being seen.

While we are here we go to the bottom of the spine at hip level and look for divots (dimples). If there are divots then it shows a weakening but not a problem. It may indicate that baby may be harder to potty train and the hips may tend to be stiff when they run as they get older but they should be fine and not have any long term issues and no reason for outside help.

Hips

With baby laying on the back, one can take baby's feet and gently bend the legs upward and then gently butterfly the knees outward and feel for clicking or cracking in the hips. This is a way to check for hip dysplasia. This does not happen often but will usually fill in and baby will have 'normal' hips as they grow and get plenty of protein into their system. If the issue is deeper into the ball and socket, baby may need to be seen by a doctor later on so keep an eye on it.

Sometimes when baby has the clicking in the hips it can also be associated with a kidney issue that makes it a little harder for them to learn to hold their urine when they are being potty trained but it is not a reason to have baby checked at this point. Just keep an eye on at baby grows and everything should be fine with it.

The hips should be smooth and at the same level. If one hip is set notably higher than the other, then baby might do well to have a gentle chiropractic adjustment in the next few weeks to have it checked.

Feet

Look for any obvious defects such as webbed toes (toes grown together), missing toes or club feet.

Webbed toes do not, usually, interfere with the way baby is going to walk or develop. There is no reason for an immediate transport or to search for medical help as baby is more in need of the bonding time with parents.

Missing toes may or may not interfere with walking so baby should be seen by a doctor within the first week or so after birth. If it is going to interfere with walking then they will want to do surgery sooner than later.

Club feet are usually caused from either genetics or environmental toxins.   It does not need to be transported immediately after birth but within the next few days afterward. Baby will require surgery in order to have a normal quality of life and be able to walk.   This is a problem that can be surgically repaired.

The next thing to look for is the color of the feet and toes. If the toes are pink (normal for the nationality) then all is well. If baby has blueness or purple then a cry should be stimulated to see if baby can pink up on it's own. A little extra oxygen might be required to help baby to maintain a healthy skin tone. Baby should also be able to hold it's color when diaper / clothing is being changed. If baby is not holding it's body heat then it will first show in the coloration in the feet. Baby's feet should never be blue.

As baby grows, the color should be watched to insure baby is getting enough oxygen and there is ample circulation.

Genitals

If baby is born in a cephalic position (head-first) then the genitals should not be swollen but if baby was born breech (bum first) then swelling is expected because the bottom is not built to withstand the pressure of the birth in that position. Therefore it is not uncommon for a baby that was born breech to have bruised genitals but they should heal in a reasonable time.

On baby girls: One wants to check to make sure that everything is intact and without bruising or with nothing protruding outside of the body. There should be an opening and it is not uncommon to have a tiny bit of blood or discharge at birth and in the few days following. Just keep clean and all should be well.

If there are any protrusions or obvious defects then baby should be seen by a care provider.

On baby boys: One will want to check for bruising and obvious signs of abnormalities. The size of the testicles should be proportionate to the size of the penis. If the testicles are very large, then one will want to pay attention to the urine in the diapers. If there are crystals or 'sediment' then baby needs to be watched for signs of kidney issues. If the testicles are swollen then it will be very uncomfortable for baby to be put into a car seat or a swing so be kind and don't ask that of him any more often than you have to until the swelling goes down.

Gently feel each side of the scrotum and see if you can feel the testicle inside. Do not 'dig' trying to find it, just gently feel.   Both testicles should be present. Genital abnormalities alone are not usually a reason to transport but warrant watching and have baby checked in the following weeks. If it is accompanied with bowel or urinary problems then baby should be seen by a care provider sooner than later.

Rectum

Upon examination the rectum should have an opening and not be sealed shut. If baby has had a bowel movement then the rectum is complete. If there is no opening then baby needs to be seen by a doctor, where surgery will probably be advised. (See Bowels section for more)

Reflexes

As a final part of the newborn exam, we take the baby's foot and firmly tickle the bottom of it with a finger nail. Baby should involuntarily flinch from the tickle along with the big toe pointing back and the other toes spreading, in a reflex known as the "Babinski Reflex".   This shows baby's reflexes are intact. Failure to respond can show that baby is very tired from a long labor or that the neurological system is not quite developed. Not a reason for transport but worth keeping an eye on.

Bowels

The bowels have a greenish-black substance called meconium that is used to hold the intestines open until they start nursing and have substance in the digestive tract.

The bowels should move within the first few hours after birth. On occasion, a baby will have a movement while still in utero causing the amniotic fluid to be stained green.   This warrants watching the baby closely for respiratory issues (See Lung section)

Once the meconium has worked it's way out of the body then the stool will turn yellow from the 'milk only' diet baby is on.

In breastfed babies, if the mother is constipated then it is very common for baby to be constipated. Usually if baby is not having regular movements then mom can eat a couple of apples per day and it will help to open babies bowels. Also if mother eats something that does not agree with baby then the baby can get loose stools or constipation. Mother needs to eat for the health and well being of baby.

There should not be blood in the stool. On occasion there might be tiny amounts now and then but if there are any significant amounts (more than just a drop or two) of blood then baby should be seen by a care provider.

Many believe that it is alright for a breastfed baby to go up to a week without a bowel movement. I find that baby is crying with a tummy ache long before that. As a rule, I like to see babies have a bowel movement in about every other diaper, for several movements per day. Babies with 2-4 movements per 24 hours tend to have less colic and are more content.

Kidneys / Bladder

Baby should urinate within the first hours after birth. If you are unsure if there is urine in the diaper (because of the polymer crystal absorption) then one can put a paper towel or a dry cloth inside the diaper that will hold onto enough of the urine to identify that there has been output.

Newborn urine should be clear and without odor. If there is blood then baby should be seen by a care provider. If the urine is brown or maple colored, this is a sign of dehydration and baby needs more water. If there is sediment like rusty colored sand then baby should be watched but there is no need for transport. Keep an eye on the diapers and make sure baby always has urine output. If any condition worsens then it is a good plan to have baby seen by your care provider.

Breastfeeding

When baby is given an opportunity to nurse within the first hour after birth, their instincts are usually good and baby will generally latch on without a lot of effort. So getting baby to the breast sooner than later is a good plan. After an hour, baby has to be taught how to nurse, so it takes more effort. Always be patient because baby has never done this before and learning to adapt.

If baby is premature then the mouth may not be big enough to latch on. At his point, baby may need to be bottle fed with mother's milk. Or a nipple shield can be used to assist with baby latching on more comfortably. Again, be patient and continue to give baby support and opportunity to figure it out.

If there was a long labor, then baby can be too tired to nurse for a while, try to get baby to latch on, even if baby does not stay latched on the baby should remember how it was done after baby wakes up. But try to wake baby every three hours to give baby a chance to eat.   It is important baby gets the colostrum, the substance the mother produces prior to her milk coming in at about 48 hours. The colostrum is loaded with everything baby needs in the first couple days after birth, oxygen and antibiotics and immune builders. When the milk comes in then it will have more fats, fluid, protein etc. which is best for baby after those first couple of days.

If baby can latch onto one side but not the other then there is a possibility that baby got it's neck a little out of place during the birth and would do well to be seen by a chiropractor with a gentle touch. Give baby a couple of days to try to figure it out by using different positions. If baby can only nurse by turning to the right then after baby eats from the left breast cradled, then baby can be put under the right arm with the feet facing moms back and baby can nurse from the right breast while still turning the neck only to the right. This would tell if the problem is with the baby's neck or a problem in the breast.

If baby's blood sugar is low then baby will latch on for a few minutes then fall asleep, sometimes in as little as 30 seconds or less. We have found that a few drops of licorice root extract will help balance baby's blood sugar and help to wake baby up so baby can stay awake to eat. Then baby will usually stay awake longer than just to nurse and fall back to sleep. It might take several days to get baby's blood sugar to regulate with this method but once baby is nursing without the licorice then the licorice should be stopped.

If the mother has had a problem in the breast such as previous infections or a mole, then the milk may not taste right and baby will reject it. If this is the case then pump some of the milk out to see if there is blood or infection in the milk.

There is an entire section on breastfeeding in the Powerfully Pregnant book if you need more help in this area.

You are finished!

If you have finished all of these checkpoints and your baby has cleared them, then you can relax.

Congratulations on your new baby! The best parts of your life are yet to come as you watch your new little one grow and change before your very eyes!

NOTES

NOTES

NOTES

NOTES

www.ingramcontent.com/pod-product-compliance
Lightning Source LLC
Chambersburg PA
CBHW050801240726
48654CB00008B/587